NAVIGATING KIDNEY DIALYSIS WITH CONFIDENCE AND CARE

Mastering And Embarking On The
Dialysis Journey For Easy Approach To
Holistic Healing

DR. WESLEY IAN

DISCLAIMER

The information in this book is not meant to replace professional medical advice, diagnosis, or treatment; rather, it is meant mainly for general informational reasons. If you have any questions about a medical problem, you should always consult your doctor or another trained health expert. Don't ever discount expert medical advice or put off getting it because of something you've read in this book.

Any negative effects or repercussions arising from the usage of the material provided herein are not the responsibility of the book's author or publisher. It should be noted by readers that the material in this book is not all-inclusive and might not address every facet of the subject. Furthermore, new research may have an impact on how health concerns are understood or treated because medical knowledge is always changing.

No particular test, treatment, method, or product mentioned in this book is endorsed or promoted by the author or publisher. The reader assumes all risk associated with using the information included in this book.

Before making any big decisions regarding your health, it's crucial to speak with a licensed healthcare provider. The relationship between a patient and their healthcare practitioner should not be replaced by this book, nor is it meant to offer medical advice.

The opinions presented in this book are the author's and may not necessarily represent those of the publisher. Any errors, omissions, or inaccuracies in the information in this book are not the responsibility of the author or publisher.

It is recommended that readers independently confirm any information contained in this book and speak with a healthcare provider about their specific medical needs and state of health.

TABLE OF CONTENTS

ABOUT THE BOOK

For those receiving kidney dialysis and those caring for them, "Navigating Kidney Dialysis with Confidence and Care" is a useful resource that offers a thorough guide to comprehending, managing, and flourishing during the dialysis journey. Using their knowledge, the author kindly provides readers with important information to help them take care of their kidneys.

To establish a rapport with readers, the book opens with a contemplative "Welcome Message" and background information on the author. The "Introduction" provides an overview of the book's goals, highlighting its function as a helpful manual for overcoming the difficulties associated with renal dialysis. The "How to Use This Guide" section guarantees that readers can get the most out of the book as a convenient companion.

The book covers the foundations, beginning with a thorough examination of renal function and the different kinds of kidney failure. In "Chapter 2: The Dialysis Process," which covers everything from preparation to the equipment used, "Understanding Kidney Dialysis" clarifies the critical role that dialysis plays in kidney care. This section demystifies the dialysis experience by providing a step-by-step procedure.

The necessity of actively participating in one's healthcare journey is emphasized: Taking Charge of Your Health". It offers helpful guidance on creating a strong support network, efficiently communicating with medical professionals, and creating reasonable health objectives. Diet and Nutrition for Dialysis Patients" discusses dietary guidelines, fluid management, and particular nutrient considerations for dialysis patients in recognition of the inseparable relationship between nutrition and health.

Lifestyle Adjustments" addresses the holistic well-being of dialysis patients and includes issues like physical activity, stress management, sleep hygiene, and mental health. Medication Management" clarifies the vital function that pharmaceuticals play in renal care, offering readers advice on how to comprehend, follow, and efficiently interact with their healthcare team.

Common Challenges and Solutions," the book addresses common challenges that arise with dialysis, such as exhaustion, emotional strain, potential complications, and troubleshooting connected to the treatment. Financial and Practical Considerations," which covers healthcare expenditures, insurance, and community resources, deftly navigates practical considerations related to daily life as well as finances. Traveling on Dialysis," the special difficulties of traveling while receiving dialysis are methodically discussed, with advice on preparation, communication with dialysis clinics, and handling medications while traveling.

"Navigating Kidney Dialysis with Confidence and Care" is an invaluable resource that empowers and teaches that receiving kidney dialysis, encouraging them to feel in control of their health journey.

CHAPTER ONE

INTRODUCTION TO KIDNEY DIALYSIS

KNOWLEDGE ABOUT DIALYSIS

Through their ability to remove waste and extra fluid from the circulation, control electrolyte balance, and produce vital hormones, the kidneys of humans are vital to the body's internal balance. On the other hand, renal failure can occur in people whose kidneys aren't functioning well enough because of a variety of medical issues. A multifaceted medical disorder, kidney failure can be divided into various categories, each with a unique etiology and effects on general health.

SYNOPSIS OF RENAL FUNCTION

It is essential to first understand the basic principles of kidney function to appreciate the significance of renal dialysis. The kidneys function as highly developed filters, drawing impurities and waste products out of the bloodstream and reabsorbing necessary components including glucose, water, and electrolytes. This complex mechanism ensures appropriate physiological functioning by keeping the body's interior environment within ideal bounds. Because of this, any decrease in kidney function has the potential to cause the body to accumulate toxic chemicals, which can lead to a variety of issues.

KIDNEY FAILURE TYPES

There are two main forms of kidney failure, which occur when the kidneys are not able to efficiently carry out their filtering functions: acute and chronic. When treated quickly, acute renal failure is usually curable and often happens rapidly.

Conversely, over a longer period, there is a progressive and permanent decline in kidney function known as chronic renal failure. End-stage renal disease (ESRD) can be brought on by chronic kidney disease (CKD), a progressive illness that calls for more sophisticated treatments like dialysis or kidney transplantation.

OVERVIEW OF DIALYSIS

Dialysis is becoming a vital therapeutic option in the field of kidney care, especially for the treatment of end-stage renal disease (ESRD). Dialysis helps to eliminate waste materials, extra fluid, and electrolytes from the bloodstream by acting as an artificial kidney substitute. When the kidneys' natural capacity to filter waste materials and maintain a proper balance of fluids and electrolytes declines to the point where the body is unable to do so, this life-sustaining process takes over. Therefore, dialysis serves as an essential lifeline for people whose kidney function is damaged, giving them the ability to manage their disease and maintain a fair quality of life.

DIALYSIS'S SIGNIFICANCE FOR KIDNEY CARE

Recognizing dialysis's ability to improve patients' general well-being, reduce kidney failure symptoms, and extend life expectancy is crucial to appreciating its significance in kidney care. Dialysis is a supportive measure that allows patients to manage their illness and carry out everyday activities, but it is not a cure for kidney failure. Additionally, dialysis plays a major role in reducing the complications of renal failure, including the build-up of harmful compounds in the body, fluid retention, and electrolyte abnormalities.

The ideas around kidney function, kidney failure kinds, and the development of dialysis are interrelated components within the larger context of renal health. Gaining a thorough comprehension of these ideas is essential to realizing the vital role that dialysis plays in the treatment and care of patients with impaired kidney function. The goal of ongoing research and developments in renal care, driven by the advancement of medical science, is to improve the quality of life for individuals affected by kidney failure by exploring alternative therapies and optimizing the effectiveness of dialysis.

CHAPTER TWO

THE PROCEDURE FOR DIALYSIS

GETTING READY FOR DIALYSIS

A thorough evaluation of the patient's health status, including a review of their medical history, a physical examination, and laboratory testing, is necessary before starting dialysis. Ensuring the patient is prepared for dialysis and taking care of any potential issues are the main goals. Before starting dialysis, patients may need to take prescribed medications, follow dietary guidelines, and monitor their fluid consumption to maintain optimal health.

PROCEDURE FOR DIALYSIS STEP-BY-STEP

Dialysis is a painstaking process designed to mimic the kidney's role in eliminating waste materials and extra fluid from the body. Vascular access is the first stage and is usually created via a central venous catheter, graft, or arteriovenous fistula. The selection of vascular access is contingent upon specific patient circumstances. The patient is linked to the dialysis machine, which functions as an artificial kidney, once access has been obtained.

Blood is taken from the patient via vascular access and goes through the dialyzer, a machine with a semipermeable membrane, during the dialysis process. This membrane replicates the kidneys' natural filtration mechanism by allowing waste materials and extra fluid to flow through. The patient's body is then given back the cleaned blood. Vital signs and other data are continuously checked during the process to guarantee the patient's safety and well-being.

EQUIPMENT & MACHINES FOR DIALYSIS

Dialysis machines are advanced medical devices that replicate the vital activities of the kidneys in an artificial environment. These devices include a dialyzer, blood pump, and other monitoring parts. The dialyzer makes it easier for substances to be exchanged between blood and dialysate, a solution that aids in the removal of waste materials, while the blood pump makes sure that blood flows through the system continuously.

The gadget also has safety measures and sirens to notify medical professionals of any problems that may arise during the treatment.

The dialysis machine is accompanied by additional equipment such as tube sets, solution bags for dialysate preparation, and needles or catheters for vascular access. Whether hemodialysis or peritoneal dialysis is ordered, the choice of equipment depends on the patient's requirements.

HOW LONG AND HOW OFTEN ARE DIALYSIS SESSIONS HELD?

Dialysis sessions differ in length and frequency based on the patient's health and the recommended course of therapy. Hemodialysis is usually done three times a week for three to five hours, though some patients may need more frequent treatments to ensure their illness is managed as best they can.

On the other hand, peritoneal dialysis is frequently carried out every day, lasting many hours per session.

Healthcare providers determine the length and frequency of dialysis depending on several factors, including the patient's overall health, reaction to prior dialysis treatments, and remaining kidney function. For dialysis patients to experience the optimum results, regular monitoring and plan modifications are essential.

CHAPTER THREE

TAKING RESPONSIBILITY FOR YOUR HEALTH

THE VALUE OF ACTIVE PARTICIPATION

Being proactive and taking control of your health entails actively participating in many facets of your well-being. The significance of taking an active role in your health management is one essential idea. This means that to preserve and enhance your general well-being, you must be knowledgeable, make thoughtful judgments, and take deliberate action. Actively engaging in your health journey, as opposed to depending exclusively on medical professionals, enables a more effective and individualized approach to wellness.

PUTTING IN PLACE A SUPPORT NETWORK

Building a strong support network is another essential part of managing your health. A support system is made up of people who are essential in motivating and helping you with your health-related activities. Family members, close friends, or even support groups with comparable health objectives might be a part of this network. Having a solid support network gives you access to emotional, psychological, and occasionally even physical help. It also creates a feeling of community and inspires you to stick with your health goals.

INTERACTING WITH HEALTHCARE PROFESSIONALS

A thorough and individualized approach to health management requires effective communication with healthcare practitioners. You can make sure that your healthcare team is fully aware of your goals, concerns, and health history by having honest and open communication with them. By working together, healthcare providers may provide more individualized guidance, well-informed recommendations, and a more efficiently executed treatment plan. You and your healthcare providers can collaborate to achieve the best possible health outcomes when you have regular, honest communication.

HAVING REASONABLE OBJECTIVES

Taking control of your health requires you to set reasonable goals. Setting unrealistic expectations might result in disappointment and even worse outcomes. You can make a successful plan by establishing goals that are both quantifiable and attainable. These goals should be specific, measurable, achievable, relevant, and time-bound (SMART). Whether your objective is to manage stress, incorporate regular exercise, or adopts a healthier diet, setting realistic goals enables you to make sustainable changes that improve your long-term well-being little by little.

Being proactive with your health entails creating a network of support, communicating effectively with medical professionals, and defining reasonable yet attainable goals.

CHAPTER FOUR

DIALYSIS PATIENTS' DIET & NUTRITION

DIALYSIS DIETARY GUIDELINES

Patients undergoing dialysis frequently experience particular difficulties in controlling their nutrition and food. The food recommendations made for dialysis patients are essential for preserving general health and controlling the side effects of renal failure. Controlling the consumption of specific nutrients is one of the main goals of maintaining appropriate nutritional balance and avoiding further renal strain.

It is usually recommended that dialysis patients closely check their protein consumption. Although protein is necessary for good health generally, eating too much of it might strain the kidneys more.

Consequently, it is advised that people see a qualified dietitian or other healthcare provider to establish a customized protein consumption that suits their unique requirements.

CONTROLLING FLUID CONSUMPTION

One of the most important dietary factors for dialysis patients is fluid management. Reduced urine flow from poor kidney function frequently makes it difficult for the body to get rid of extra fluid. As a result, dialysis patients must carefully control how much fluid they consume to avoid fluid overload, which can result in consequences including hypertension, edema, and cardiovascular problems.

Patients are usually recommended to restrict their fluid intake, which includes keeping an eye on the foods and drinks they consume as well as items high in water content, such as fruits, vegetables, and soups. Furthermore, methods like occasionally freezing some liquids and eating them as ice chips might reduce thirst without breaking fluid limitations.

NEEDS FOR NUTRIENTS

To stay as healthy as possible, dialysis patients need to be very mindful of the total amount of nutrients they consume. In addition to controlling protein and fluids, they must make sure that necessary vitamins and minerals are ingested in sufficient amounts. Minerals like potassium and phosphorus as well as water-soluble vitamins like the B vitamins are frequently lost during dialysis.

Healthcare providers may suggest particular supplements or dietary changes to treat these issues. Dialysis patients, for example, need to watch how much phosphorus they eat since too much of it in the blood can lead to problems with their bones and cardiovascular systems. It's also critical to keep an eye on potassium levels because low kidney function can raise potassium levels, which may result in heart problems.

PARTICULAR THINGS TO THINK ABOUT FOR DIALYSIS PATIENTS

Dialysis patients may have extra obstacles and things to think about while making food decisions. For instance, limits on specific fruits and vegetables that are high in potassium could be required. Analyzing salt consumption is also essential for controlling blood pressure and fluid balance.

Furthermore, dialysis patients frequently prioritize controlling their weight and taking care of any nutritional issues. Dietary techniques must be used to treat the accidental weight loss that some people may have to stop future issues. Together with medical specialists, routine nutritional status evaluations can assist in customizing dietary advice to meet the unique requirements of each patient.

The dietary guidelines for dialysis adopt a comprehensive approach, focusing on individualized nutrition regimens that take particular considerations, fluid management, protein consumption, and nutrient requirements into account. Following these recommendations is essential for improving the general health and quality of life of those coping with kidney failure and dialysis.

CHAPTER FIVE

MODIFICATIONS TO LIFESTYLE

EXERCISE AND PHYSICAL ACTIVITY

A healthy lifestyle must include both regular exercise and physical activity. There are several advantages to physical activity for both the body and the mind. It increases cardiovascular health, strengthens and stretches muscles, and aids in maintaining a healthy weight. Additionally, exercise plays a key role in preventing numerous chronic illnesses, such as heart disease, diabetes, and obesity.

In addition to its physical benefits, regular physical activity lowers stress, anxiety, and depression, which in turn improves mental health. It encourages the body's natural mood enhancers, endorphins, to be released, which improves one's attitude on life. Including a variety of cardio, strength, and flexibility activities in one's program will help one feel more fit and energetic overall.

SLEEP MANAGEMENT

Sustaining the highest possible level of health and well-being requires getting enough good sleep. Immune system performance, memory consolidation, emotional control, and other physiological and cognitive processes all depend on sleep. Effective sleep management mostly involves establishing a regular sleep schedule and establishing a sleep-friendly atmosphere. It entails sticking to a regular sleep schedule, making sure your bedroom is calm and dark, and avoiding stimulants like caffeine right before bed. Making good sleep hygiene a priority will greatly enhance the quality of sleep, which will enhance overall cognitive function, mood stability, and focus.

TECHNIQUES FOR REDUCING STRESS

In the fast-paced world of today, stress management is essential for mental and physical well-being. A variety of stress-reduction strategies can assist people in managing the difficulties of life. For example, practicing mindfulness and meditation can help one become more aware of the present moment, which reduces stress and improves emotional health. Other useful methods for reducing stress include yoga, progressive muscle relaxation, and deep breathing exercises. Taking up hobbies, going outside, and keeping a good work-life balance are some ways to reduce stress. Since chronic stress has been connected to a wide range of health problems, such as digestive illnesses, mental health disorders, and cardiovascular diseases, it is imperative to develop good coping techniques.

SOCIAL AND EMOTIONAL WELL-BEING

Two essential components of a happy existence are strong social ties and emotional stability. Significantly influencing emotional wellness is the development and maintenance of relationships with friends, family, and communities. A sense of community is fostered by social support, which also lessens feelings of loneliness and improves general well-being. Emotional resilience is influenced by open communication and honest emotional expression. Acquiring the ability to identify and control one's emotions, or emotional intelligence, is a crucial life skill for overcoming obstacles. Maintaining emotional well-being also requires cultivating a good outlook, practicing appreciation, and partaking in joyful activities. Maintaining a balanced and emotionally fulfilling existence requires finding a way to combine social engagements with personal leisure.

CHAPTER SIX

MEDICATION ADMINISTRATION
COMPREHENDING DRUGS

Effective medication management requires a thorough understanding of drugs. It entails having a thorough understanding of the prescription drug's intended use, dosage, and administration. Patients need to understand how their medications work, how the body reacts to them, and the desired results. This knowledge encourages a sense of control and involvement in the patient journey by enabling people to make educated decisions regarding their care. For patients to actively engage in conversations with their healthcare professionals and make sure that their treatment plans are tailored to their requirements and objectives, they must be literate in pharmacology.

FOLLOWING MEDICATION SCHEDULE

Following a prescribed medication schedule is essential to getting the best possible therapeutic results.

Maintaining therapeutic levels in the body requires consistency in taking drugs at the recommended times and doses. Disregarding the suggested timetable may impair the treatment's efficacy, resulting in less-than-ideal outcomes or, in certain situations, treatment failure. People can stay on top of their medication regimen by creating routine and using tools like pill organizers or medication reminder apps. A successful treatment plan also depends on effective communication with healthcare practitioners to resolve any issues or worries about adherence and look into other options.

POSSIBLE SIDE CONSEQUENCES

Patients must be able to make educated decisions about their care by being aware of the possible negative consequences of the medications they take. Adverse effects of medications can range in severity and duration, from minor to severe. Patients should know when to seek emergency medical treatment and be aware of frequent side effects as well as uncommon but significant problems. It is essential to have open lines of contact with medical professionals about any adverse effects encountered while receiving therapy. This balances the advantages and disadvantages of the recommended therapy and permits prompt modifications to the drug schedule or investigation of substitute options. The overall safety and efficacy of the medication are improved by taking a proactive approach to side effect management.

INTERACTING WITH YOUR MEDICAL TEAM

A key component of good drug management is good communication between patients and their medical team. Healthcare professionals can learn about a patient's experience with prescribed medications, including any difficulties or worries about side effects or adherence, by having an honest and open discussion with them. Patients should actively engage in conversations regarding their treatment plan, offering input on how it affects their day-to-day activities and general state of health. Regular follow-up sessions and proactive communication channels, such as secure messaging or telemedicine consultations, provide continual monitoring and adjustment of the treatment plan as needed. Establishing a cooperative rapport with the medical staff fosters a patient-focused methodology, guaranteeing that the medication management plan corresponds with the person's distinct requirements, inclinations, and objectives.

CHAPTER SEVEN

TYPICAL PROBLEMS AND THEIR FIXES

HANDLING FATIGUE

People often struggle with fatigue in a variety of spheres of life, and it can be more severe for those receiving medical care or dealing with long-term health issues. Managing fatigue becomes important in the context of healthcare, particularly for patients receiving dialysis treatments. Dialysis can be physically taxing, which can leave one feeling worn out and exhausted. Due to the lengthy nature of dialysis treatments, which can interfere with daily activities and leave patients feeling exhausted, patients frequently experience weariness.

The use of individualized treatment programs is one way to manage weariness in dialysis patients. Dialysis regimens can be customized to fit a patient's tastes and lifestyle to reduce interruptions and maximize energy. To give patients greater flexibility and convenience and, eventually, lessen the impact of fatigue on their daily lives, healthcare providers may also investigate the usage of cutting-edge technologies or home-based dialysis choices.

MANAGING EMOTIONAL STRESS

Coping with long-term medical illnesses and therapies always leads to emotional stress. Dialysis patients frequently struggle with emotional issues including loneliness, melancholy, or worry. Emotional strain can be caused by the repeated nature of dialysis sessions and their impact on one's quality of life, which can affect the patient as well as their support system.

An all-encompassing approach to patient treatment is necessary to address emotional distress. The mental health of dialysis patients can be greatly enhanced by including mental health services in the entire treatment plan. Patients can share their stories and get advice from psychosocial interventions, counseling services, and support groups. Additionally, encouraging open communication between patients and healthcare professionals' helps to establish a setting in which emotional issues can be recognized and successfully handled, supporting a more all-encompassing approach to treatment.

HANDLING POSSIBLE DIFFICULTIES

Dialysis patients are vulnerable to several consequences, from vascular access problems to infections. Ensuring the safety and well-being of dialysis patients requires preventing and treating these possible consequences. Effective management greatly depends on routine monitoring and early detection of problems.

Putting in place thorough education initiatives for patients and healthcare professionals is one way to address this. Providing healthcare workers with up-to-date knowledge of dialysis technology and treatment protocols might improve their capacity to recognize and rapidly manage possible issues. In addition, patients are empowered to actively participate in their treatment and take preventive action when they are taught self-care techniques and how to spot early warning signs of consequences. Working together, patients and healthcare professionals can take a proactive approach to controlling and minimizing any issues that may arise from dialysis.

TROUBLESHOOTING PROBLEMS WITH DIALYSIS

Dialysis-related complications can emerge owing to several circumstances, including mechanical failures, access challenges, or poor clearance of toxins. Effective troubleshooting is essential to reducing treatment process interruptions and guaranteeing dialysis session efficacy.

The creation of comprehensive training programs for medical personnel providing dialysis therapy is one practical answer. Giving them thorough instruction on handling frequent technological problems and crises gives them the tools they need to solve problems quickly. Furthermore, equipping patients with rudimentary troubleshooting skills improves their capacity to recognize and convey problems during or in between dialysis treatments.

CHAPTER EIGHT

PRACTICAL AND FINANCIAL ASPECTS TO TAKE INTO ACCOUNT

MANAGING MEDICAL EXPENSES

Navigating the complicated world of healthcare expenditures is one of the most important parts of managing practical and financial considerations. Medical costs can put a heavy strain on both individuals and families in the modern world. It is crucial to comprehend the nuances of healthcare costs, including hospital bills, prescription drugs, and outpatient services. To avoid any financial surprises, it is imperative to take the initiative to actively seek clear information on the expenses of medical procedures and treatments.

PROTECTION FROM INSURANCE

Getting the right kind of insurance is essential to protecting one's finances. One of the most important factors in reducing the effects of medical costs is health insurance. It is essential to read insurance policies thoroughly and be aware of the deductibles, co-payments, and coverage limitations. People should evaluate their healthcare needs and select insurance policies that meet their demands. Insurance coverage should be reviewed and updated regularly to make sure it stays applicable to evolving situations and acts as a safety net in the event of unforeseen medical issues.

USEFUL ADVICE FOR EVERYDAY LIFE

Practical and financial factors are not limited to healthcare; they also include other facets of daily life. Individuals and families can preserve their financial stability by implementing sensible spending habits, tracking their expenses, and creating budgets.

One of the most important steps in financial planning is creating a realistic budget that takes savings, discretionary spending, and necessities into consideration. Long-term financial well-being is also influenced by investigating cost-saving options and developing sound spending habits.

Community Resources and Support Communities frequently provide a multitude of resources and networks of support that can ease practical and financial difficulties. Assistance with housing, food, utility bills, and other necessities may be available via neighborhood associations, charitable organizations, and government initiatives. Making ties within the community enables people to use these resources and take advantage of the assistance offered. Additionally, neighborhood networks and support groups can provide practical and emotional support, fostering a sense of camaraderie in overcoming barriers linked to health and finances.

Taking into account practical and financial factors requires a thorough strategy that takes into account community resources, healthcare expenditures, insurance coverage, and workable daily living practices. People can better handle the challenges of managing their finances and general well-being by actively interacting with these issues.

CHAPTER NINE

DIALYSIS TRAVELERS

PLANNING FOR TRAVEL

To guarantee a seamless and stress-free experience when traveling for dialysis, careful planning is essential. Dialysis patients must organize their travel arrangements well in advance to fit their treatment routine. This entails taking into account the length of the journey, how frequently dialysis sessions are held, and how easily accessible the dialysis facilities are once at the destination. Travelers should speak with their medical team to determine whether the trip is feasible and to get the required medical clearance.

INTERACTING WITH DIALYSIS FACILITIES

For dialysis patients traveling, it is essential to communicate effectively with the dialysis centers. To schedule treatment appointments, travelers should get in touch with possible dialysis facilities before setting out on their travels. It's critical to communicate clearly about dialysis medications, medical data, and any special needs. Giving the destination dialysis center comprehensive details on a patient's medical history and current treatment plan helps them better prepare for the patient's arrival and guarantees continuity of care.

TAKING CARE OF DRUGS WHILE TRAVELING

Taking care of prescriptions while traveling, particularly for dialysis patients, calls for considerable thought and preparation. Enough prescription medication, together with any over-the-counter medications and supplements, must be packed. Travelers should arrange their meds safely and conveniently, taking into account things like meal plans and time zone shifts. In case of an emergency, it is also a good idea to have a documented list of all the medications you take, their dosages, and the doctor who prescribed them.

MAKING SURE YOUR TRIP IS EASY

People on dialysis should acquaint themselves with the medical facilities and services offered at their destination to have a seamless travel experience. A sense of security can be enhanced by learning about the area's emergency services, researching neighboring dialysis centers, and having a backup plan in case of unanticipated medical problems. A comfortable and accommodating travel experience can also be ensured by disclosing to airline and hotel staff any special medical concerns, such as the need for medicine refrigeration or aid with mobility.

To guarantee a smooth vacation experience, dialysis patients must plan carefully, communicate effectively with healthcare providers, carefully monitor their meds, and take proactive measures. Dialysis patients who prioritize their health and well-being can confidently travel to new places by taking care of these issues.